"Dark Eye Circles Gone

by Charles Silverman N.D.

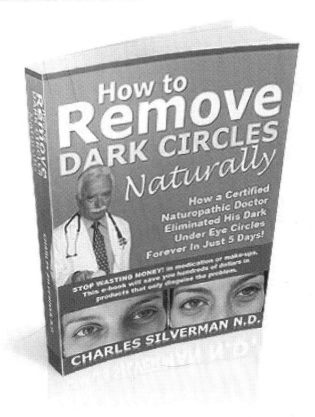

About

Charles Silverman N.D., a Naturalist and Herbalist since 1979, is the author of the Home Made Medicine e-book and the www.HomeMadeMedicine.com Web site. Charles lives in Miami, FL and has dedicated a major part of his life to the preparation of natural remedies and natural products to help people with allergies
and chemical intolerance. He has traveled around the world from Canada, Germany, France, and India to the mountains of Peru and Argentina (South America) researching and studying the different domestic species of herbs and plants.   His articles are published on several web sites like ezinearticles.com and naturalhealthweb.com and he is regularly interviewed by various publications and
newspapers like the Montgomery News of Alabama. All his knowledge has been transferred to his web site and now to this amazing book, that takes advantage of the latest technology in order to bring you the most complete guide for home healing ever made.

WWW.CHARLES-SILVERMAN.COM

Be curious always! For knowledge will not acquire you: you must acquire it.

~ Sudie Back ~

Disclaimer

Information in this book is provided for informational purposes and is not meant to substitute for the advice of your physician or health care professional. You should not use this information to diagnose or treat a health problem or disease, nor to prescribe any medication. You should read all product packaging and labels carefully. If you have or suspect that you have a medical condition, promptly contact your health care provider.

Remember that some herbs if used often may produce some minor irritations or stomach upsets. If you are allergic to ragweed or any other plant, consult your physician before taking any herbal remedy.

How to use this report

This report (if used correctly) can help you get rid of your dark circles under the eyes. To get test result using the e-book you must first identify the cause of your dark circles. Don't worry; I will help you recognize your problem as w move along, but I must insist that you or your doctors are the ones that must diagnose the underlying condition causing your dark circles.

Once you have found the source of your dark circles you can start using the remedies recommended for that particular illness and you may combine ther with the Nutrition Section and the common Home remedies for Dark Circles Section.

Next you should read the section on special Dark circles remedy and make the 5 day dark circle remedy recipe.

You don't have to use all of the remedies and herbs, choose the ones that go with your primary illness.

Don't forget to use the information in the "Do Not Do This" List to remove from your life style the habits that normally contribute to developing dark circles.

Finally you should read the section on immune system and make one of the immune system recipes.

At the end of the report you will find a list of herbs, vitamins and minerals used throughout this e-book to treat dark circles. Read it very carefully, since these herbs are used for dark circles and many other conditions.

Introduction: a short personal story

It was five years ago I was invited to speak in a convention on natural therapies, in Miami; I was so honored and thrilled. My wife and some friends were going to be there, so we decided to make it a fun evening by going to dinner after the convention.

I spend a week writing what I was going to say in front of many of my colleges, this was very important to me and I wanted to make a good impression. But during the days prior to the event I started to be preoccupied about my appearance, not because I look bad, after all I work out every other day; the reason for my worries were my dark circles under my eyes, I have a fairly white complexion and when I'm under attack by this shiners I look almost dead.

So the day came and sure enough I found myself in front of the mirror staring at my own face, there they were, right under my eyes again. If it was not for my tuxedo, I would have looked like Mike Tyson just had a boxing practice with my face. I was really disturbed and angry, I knew I had to do something quick, but did not know what.

So I did what no man would ever do, I cover my dark circles with my wife's makeup. I did not care I had to look good, this was my night. After a few minutes in the bathroom applying a skin tone base, that Anny handed me, I was satisfied by the outcome, it was not perfect but they were not as noticeable as before.

I was very nervous as I walked to the small stage prepared for the speakers; a microphone and a very bright light were waiting for me. As I started to speak I saw all those people listening to me, it was very scary, everybody was looking at me in silence and this made me even more self-conscious. As the minutes went by the light and my tuxedo, were conspiring to make me perspire. I noticed how my forehead was getting damp. Eventually sweat started to roll down from the sides of my head, this made me very nervous, but I was able to finish without anybody noticing anything.

Once I finished I walked back to my table, as I sat down my wife immediately said to me ¨Honey you are sweating¨, I quickly took my handkerchief and wiped my face down, even the back of my neck, which it was wet too. That's when I saw that all of the makeup that I so carefully putted on, was now smeared all over this piece of cloth.

I went to the washroom and in there my fears were confirmed, my dark circles under the eyes were in the front row again, what a nightmare, I looked sad and older.

A few days after the convention I received the photos taken during that night, I looked tired, old and sad. This was a turning point for me, because I realized that I had to do something. I'm a Naturopathic Doctor that helps people be healthier, yet I look ill.

That same day I started doing my research, looking for an answer, a solution to this problem.

Five years later I can say that I know everything there is to know about dark circles under the eyes and here is my experience. Everything I was able to learn I transferred to this report, to help you get rid of your dark circles, like I did.

What are dark circles under the eyes?

The medical term for dark rings under the eyes is 'infraorbital hyperpigmentaion' or 'infraorbital pigmentation' knowing these terms is not necessary, but it helps to know what we are up against. Basically, Dark circles around the eyes are simply blood passing through veins just below the surface of the skin. They worsen with age, when tired, during menstruation or pregnancy; they sometimes are a symptom of an underlying medical problem or body deficiency.

Dark circles under the eyes are noticeable because the   layer of skin (and underlying fat) are thinnest at this point compared to other parts of your body, so the deep purple color of the blood in the vessels shows through. The lighter your skin color, the more the color from the blood vessels shows through. We have more blood vessels per area in the head (one of the reason a head wound produces so much more blood compared to cuts in other parts of the body). So not only does the thinner skin allow more of the purple from the blood vessels show through, there are more blood vessels, proportionally, to be seen.

What causes Dark circles?

Dark circles under or around the eyes can be caused by many different factors. The following are the most common causes and the remedies you should use for each case, however, please note that a

combination of cases could be affecting you and causing Dark Circles under your eyes. You must first identify your own cause or causes whichever it may be.

HEREDITY

One cause of dark circles under the eyes is genes, for many this will be the main reason they have this ugly condition. If someone in your family has dark circles, chances are you will get them as well.   Like varicose veins, dark circles under the eyes are usually an inherited trait. If you have dark circles, there is a good chance that others in your family also have them.

The skin under the eye is very thin; when blood passes through the large veins close to the surface of the skin it can produce a bluish tint. The more transparent your skin, also an inherited trait, the darker the circles appear.

Most people who find out that their circles are inherited become frustrated, because most professionals will tell them that they must be surgically removed.

This is not entirely true; you see one of the new vogues in plastic surgery is laser treatment for dark circles; this is starting to bring big money to plastic surgeons, they use Photo rejuvenation, Laser Resurfacing, or a vascular laser to remove the dark under the eyes.

The truth is; not everyone that has dark circles needs surgery to remove them, sure in some very severe cases it may be the only way to go, but before you open your wallet, shouldn't you try the natural way first?

Don't put yourself under the knife yet; read this entire report use the remedies we recommend you will be amazed by the results.

There is much misinformation out there, don't put your body through a Chemical Peel until you know for sure that is the only way to getting rid of your dark circles.

Even if your dark circles are inherited, natural remedies will help.

How?

You must understand this, you don't just inherit the dark circles; you inherit the condition that causes them. This means that if your family is genetically pre dispose to have liver problems you probably will too and as we will see later on, liver problems are one of the reasons dark circles appear. Simple... right? Then why didn't anybody told you that before?   The answer is also simple, by simplifying their answer doctors leave you with only one alternative, get them surgically removed.

Now you know better.

First you most find out what is causing the dark circles, then you must choose a natural approach, if that didn't work, you can start considering a more invasive treatment.

Some of the cases I have seen were solved by simple changes in life style, this are the same people that were told that their dark circles were inherited and that they should ether learn to live with them or have them surgically removed.

EXPOSURE TO THE SUN

This is one of those myths that I never understood and always disagree on, most people will tell you that exposure to sunlight, especially during the summer months; can cause a higher-than-normal level of skin pigmentation (melanin) under the eyes. People get sun tans because exposure to the sun increases the natural pigmentation of the skin and draws that pigmentation to the surface and they believe that somehow this causes dark circles to appear. In my experience this is totally wrong, the sun does increase the pigmentation of the skin, however, that has nothing to do with your dark circles.

Dark circles are blood vessels showing through the thin skin in the eye area and I know for sure that in the summer time when my dark circles were really bad I was able to disguise them by getting a tan on my face. This principle is totally wrong in my book.

So, now we know that dark circles are blood vessels showing through the skin and that sun does not causes them, but let me clarify something, this does not mean that the darker your skin the less noticeable your dark circles are going to be.

I'm sure you are aware of the fact that people from India have a tendency to develop dark circles, if you observe closely you will notice that this is true and as you know they also have a dark complexion.

This proves that even if your skin is dark; you can have very noticeable dark circles around your eyes. Sun tan can help but will not make then fade away completely.

The skin around the eyes is very thin, transparent and fragile, raising the pigmentation may help disguise the dark vessels underneath, however a disguise is not a treatment, it accomplishes only a temporary cover up of the condition.

ALLERGIES, ASTHMA and ECZEMA

Now we're talking about some real culprits of dark circles under eyes, but these causes actually has several sub categories, because there are many allergies that affect us and most of them cause dark circles. Any condition that causes your eyes to itch or your sinus to congest can contribute to darker circles under the eyes.

Rubbing or scratching the skin can damage the fragile capillaries, remember that capillaries are very thin blood vessels, if you scratch, or even stroke too much this area you could rupture these vessels and when that happens your skin darkens. Sinus congestions also contribute to dark circles, the pressure in the sinus or the strain generated by constantly blown your nose, will cause the capillaries to rupture, thus giving you the already famous "allergic shiners",

Hay fever

Sufferers particularly will notice under-eye "smudges" during the height of the allergy season. Hay fever is a common nasal allergy to airborne substances such as pollens or molds and the term has also been used for other allergies such as to animal dander. It is very common with an estimated 35 million Americans with pollen allergies alone. Hay fever is also known as "allergic rhinitis".

Symptoms are often similar to a cold with runny nose, tearing, sneezing and so on. Another possibility that must be ruled out is asthma, but we will deal with this later. There are also numerous subtypes of hay fever and it is desirable to determine exactly what is causing the allergy. One key factor is whether symptoms are seasonal, especially for pollen allergies, or year-round as for some other types of allergies all of which contribute to developing dark circles.

A balanced, nutrient-rich, noncongesting diet is best. Eat plenty of fresh fruits and vegetables; whole grains like rice, millet and oats; legumes, both cooked and sprouted; some raw seeds and nuts (but not peanuts); and some lean, clean fish and poultry proteins. Avoid foods that tend to promote congestion. These include breads and baked goods, cheese and dairy foods, sugar and refined flours and most packaged or processed foods.

- Common allergic foods are dairy products, eggs, wheat, sugar, soy products, yeast, peanuts and citrus fruits. Eliminate these from your diet for two or three weeks to see whether the symptoms improve.

- Salmon and flounder contain oil that is considered anti-inflammatory and to maximize the result they should be consumed two or three times a week if possible, you can also take them in gel-capsule form.

- SHILAJIT is an herb with over sixty years of clinical research which have shown that shilajit has positive effects on humans. It increases longevity, improves memory and cognitive ability, reduces allergies and respiratory problems and reduces stress.

- Don't take alcohol, sugar, caffeine and nicotine, these substances interfere and stress the immune system.

- Primrose oil contains gamma-linolenic acid (GLA), which has inti-inflammatory and anti-allergic effects. Take a dose of primrose oil that provides 250 milligrams of gamma-linolenic acid three times a day.

- Sulfur, in the form of methylsulfonylmethane (MSM), may help decrease an allergic reaction. Take 500milligrams 2 or 3 times a day.

- The B-complex vitamins, especially B6 (Pyridoxine) and pantothenic acid, aid in the processing of food amino acids. They also support the function of the adrenal glands, which is important in the control of allergies.   Take 100 milligrams of vitamin b6 and 250 milligrams pantothenic acid twice a day between meals, for up to five days.

• Taking 1,000 milligrams vitamin C, plus an equal amount of bioflavonoids three times a day, six weeks before the hay-fever season arrives.

Hay Fever Preventive Tincture

½ tsp. Siberian ginseng root tincture.
½ tsp. nettle leaves tincture.
½ tsp. elder flowers tincture.
½ tsp. peppermint leaves tincture.
Combine ingredients; Take a half a dropperful at least 5 times a day. Start the preventive treatment at the begging of the season.

Dust mite

Dust mite allergy is an allergy to a microscopic organism that lives in the dust commonly found in all dwellings and workplaces. Dust mites are perhaps the most common cause of perennial allergic rhinitis.

Dust mite allergy usually produces symptoms similar to pollen allergy and also can produce symptoms of asthma.

The list of symptoms mentioned in various sources for Dust mite allergies includes:

- Year-round symptoms - not seasonal like most pollen or mold allergies
- Sneezing
- Runny nose
- Blocked nose
- Coughing
- Postnasal drip
- Itching eyes
- Itching nose
- Itching throat

- Dark circles under the eyes (Allergic shiners)
- Nose rubbing
- Allergic salute (persistent upward nose rubbing)
- Watering eyes
- Conjunctivitis
- Red-rimmed eyes
- Swollen eyes
- Crusting of eyelids

Along with pollens from trees, grasses and weeds, molds are an important cause of seasonal allergic rhinitis. People allergic to molds may have symptoms from spring to late fall. The mold season often peaks from July to late summer. Unlike pollens, molds may persist after the first killing frost. Some can grow at subfreezing temperatures, but most become dormant. Snow cover lowers the outdoor mold count dramatically but does not kill molds. After the spring thaw, molds thrive on the vegetation that has been killed by the winter cold.

The most common symptoms associated with exposure to certain molds include the following: nasal stuffiness, eye irritation, wheezing, aggravation of asthma, cold/flu like symptoms, rashes, fever, shortness of breath, inability to concentrate, fatigue, Dark circles under the eyes (Allergic shiners), Crusting of eyelids, Swollen eyes, sometimes lung infections and Red-rimmed eyes. As you can see these allergies punish the eye area quite a bit.

Homemade Nasal Inhaler

¼ tsp. coarse salt.
5 drops of eucalyptus essential oil.
Place salt in a small plastic squeeze bottle with lid, add the oil. The salt will soak up the oil; let it rest for two or three hours. Remove the lid and inhale deeply as you squeeze the bottle, pushing the air only into your nostril.

This remedy clears the sinus and allows easier breathing, which reduces the pressure that can cause dark circles.

Sinus Congestion Tea

1 tsp. yarrow flowers.
1 tsp. elder flowers.
1 tsp. peppermint leaves.
Pour boiling water over herbs and steep for at least 20 minutes in a covered container. Strain out the herbs. Drink the tea a few times a day.

Dermatitis or Eczema

Dermatitis is an inflammatory skin condition that produces blisters, redness, scaling, flaking, thickening, weeping, crusting, color changes and itching that can be very annoying. Many times Dermatitis is allergic in nature mainly by coming in contact with different materials, chemicals or plants, such as, rubber, latex, perfumes, gold, silver, poison ivy, soap, cosmetics etc.

People with thin dry skin are prone to develop dermatitis and other skin conditions.   Another cause of dermatitis is sensitivity or allergy to some foods. Studies have shown that people with low stomach acid are sensitive to some types of foods thus making them prone to develop some kind of skin disorder.

People suffering from dermatitis are sensitive to some of the items listed above and should be mindful of their condition and avoid contact with any irritant. Prolonged exposure to the materials may worsen the symptoms and cause the dermatitis to spread.

If you suspect or your doctor has diagnosed your dark circles as being cause by eczema you can try some excellent home remedies I have recommended for years, below you will find some very useful natural preparations you can make to treat eczema.

Skin wash

Mix the following ingredients:
1 tsp. comfrey root.
1 tsp. white oak bark.
1 tsp. slippery elm bark.
2 cups of water.
Boil for 35 minutes use it to wash the affected area.

- Vitamin B complex is needed for healthy skin.

- Take Biotin pills is essential to prevent dermatitis.

TIP: Did you know that foods containing raw eggs prevent

biotin from being absorbed?

- Put Vitamin E on the affected area it calms the itching.

- Take Zinc orally and apply it directly on the dermatitis.

- Shark cartilage reduces inflammation.

- Use a lotion made out of blueberry leaves this is proven to be fantastic relieving inflammation of dermatitis.

- Rue contains flavonoids needed for inflammation reduction.

- Drink chamomile it helps with inflammation.

- Make a paste mixing goldenseal root powder, Vitamin E oil and honey apply directly on the skin, this speeds up healing.

Skin Infection fighting tea.
Make a tea mixing:
1 tsp. burdock root.
1 tsp. Oregon grape root.
1 tsp. echinacea root.
1 tsp. yellow dock root.
3 cups of water.
Boil for 20 minutes, drink ½ a cup a day.

- Do not eat the following: eggs, peanuts, wheat, dairy products, sugar, strawberries and flour.

- Use a cream made with tea tree oil. It helps to kill microbes and it's a natural antiseptic.

Dermatitis skin treatment

½ pau d'arco bark tincture.
½ goldenseal root tincture.
8 drops tea tree essential oil.
8 drops chamomile essential oil.
½ cups of olive oil.
½   ounce of dried comfrey leaves.
½   ounce dried calendula flowers.
½   ounce of pure beeswax.
4 drops lavender essential oil.
Heat the olive oil with comfrey and calendula in it for about 2 hours without making the oil boil. Strain while warm, add beeswax and heat enough to melt it. Add essential oils and tinctures and stir well. Apply as needed over the skin.

• A very powerful herb used to treat psoriasis and dermatitis is sarsaparilla, as publish in the 1940's by the New England journal of medicine "dramatically" successful in treating these types of conditions.

Skin Poultice.

A poultice is very helpful prepared as follows:
1 tablespoon of dried coneflower flowers.
1 tablespoon of hyssop flowers.
1 tablespoon of goldenrod flowers.
1 tablespoon of dried sunflower petals.
Mix ingredients and soak them with boiling water, let cool, place between gauze and apply on the skin, re moistening as needed.

Natural Antiseptic spray

1/8 tsp. lemon essential oil.
1/8 tsp. tea tree essential oil.
½ ounce goldenseal tincture.
½ ounce Oregon grape root tincture or barberry bark tincture.
1 ½ ounces aloe vera.
Mix all the ingredients and shake well every day for a week. Place liquid in a spray bottle, shake well before use.

• Studies done in France on the herbs milk thistle and gotu kola have shown compounds that greatly improve psoriasis and dermatitis. These herbs are being used in French hospitals in the form of salve and as an injection and people in that country have used them for many years to cure leprosy.

• Licorice is a very powerful herb to reduce the inflammation and stress related to many types of dermatitis.

• The compound gamma linoleic acid (GLA) found in primrose oil reduces inflammation of the skin better then cortisone, as shown in a study done on 100 people.

Dermatitis tea

½ tsp. sarsaparilla root.
½ tsp. licorice root.
½ tsp. burdock root.
½ tsp. pau d'arco bark.
½ tsp. bupleurum root.
3 cups of water.
Simmer for 10 minutes and steep for another 10 minutes. Strain and drink 3 cups a day.

• Take 500 milligrams of red clover 3 times a day.
Asthma is also known to cause dark circles under the eyes, if you regularly suffer from asthma attacks you can be sure your dark circles are due to this respiratory disease.

TIP: Medication used to treat high blood pressure can cause life threatening complications in people with asthma.

Asthma is a very common respiratory disease. It affects the trachea and bronchial tubes by becoming inflamed and plugged with mucus. This causes the airways to narrow restricting the amount of air going to the lungs and makes it very difficult to breathe. Asthma can occur in anyone but is very common in children and early adulthood. Typical symptoms of an asthma attack are coughing, wheezing, tight chest, difficulty breathing.

There are two types of asthma: allergic and non-allergic.   Some of the allergens that can trigger an asthma attack are chemicals, drugs, smoke, dust, food additives, pollution, mold, etc. Non allergic asthma can be cause by anxiety, exercise, dry or humid weather, fear, laughing, stress etc.

The rate, in which asthma attacks, has increased in the past few years is alarming, especially in children. Scientists believe that, there is a strong link between contamination in the air we breathe and asthma.

Evidence suggests that, the percentage of people who live in big cities and have asthma attacks is far greater than those of people who live in rural areas, however, these may not be the only reasons, genetic, food additives, toxins etc.

Children with asthma also develop dark circles and modern medicine can offer very little to children with asthma. Most drugs can only produce a temporary effect. Herbs in the other hand can be very helpful not only reducing attacks but also strengthening the lungs and immune system.

TIP: Did you know that aspirin, Advil, chemotherapy and antibiotics can cause asthma attacks?

- Vitamin B6 and Vitamin B12 are very important nutrients to treat asthma decreasing the inflammation in the lungs.

- Vitamin C is needed to fight infection, increase the amount of oxygen and reduce inflammation.

- Use ginkgo biloba, this herb contains ginkgolide B which is very helpful. Some studies indicate that ginkgo biloba reduces the frequency of asthma attacks.

- Mullein oil is used to fight respiratory congestion is very important to make it as a tea for faster results.

- Pau d'arco is a natural antibiotic and reduces inflammation.

- In china a powerful mixture of herbs called Shuan Huang Lian is being used in hospitals to treat respiratory illness, very important to use this herb in asthma and acute bronchitis.

If exercise triggers asthma attacks, cut back the amount of salt in your diet and take 2,000 mg. of Vitamin C one hour before your workout.

- Eat salmon 3 times a week or take salmon oil capsules.

Asthma Tea

Make a tea using:
2 tsp. powdered Indian root.
2 tsp. granulated Echinacea root.
2 tsp. elecampane root.
2 cups of water.
Mix all ingredients and let them set for 2 hours.

To improve breathing

Make a tea with:

1 quart boiling water.
1 tsp. chamomile flowers.
1 tsp. Echinacea root.
1 tsp. mullein leaves.
1 tsp. passionflower leaves.
Mix herbs and pour boiling water over them, steep for 20 minutes, strain and give ½ a cup a day.

Throat spray for asthma attacks
(This remedy is used as many asthmatic inhalers).

1 tsp. ginkgo leaves (tincture form).
5 drops chamomile essential oil.
1/4 cup of water.
Mix all the liquids and store them in a spray or pump bottle, use as needed, this remedy keeps airways clear and dilated.

• A very tasteful herb for children is Lemon verbena tea. This herb reduces wheezing and doctors recommend it in South America.

Chinese preparation remedy

1 tsp. magnolia flowers.
1 tsp. rehmannia root.
½ tsp. don quai root.
3 cups of water.
Boil all ingredients and simmer for 15 minutes, remove from heat and steep for another 15 minutes, strain and give 1 cup a day.

• In recent studies, scientists in Germany discovered that onion contains some compounds that are very helpful with asthma. Drink 1 glass of onion juice a day.

• Jamaican Dogwood is a strong pain reliever, sedative and antispasmodic. It is very helpful for muscular back pain, asthma, menstrual pain, insomnia, toothaches and nervous conditions.

Medication

Any medication that you are taking that causes blood vessels to dilate can cause circles under the eyes to darken. Because the skin under the eyes is very delicate, any increase blood flow shows through the skin.

Medication like doxepine changes sleep architecture, the ongoing sedation and anticholinergic activity, as well as, water retention and sodium exchange changes, that this drug creates can contribute to getting dark circles.

The herb Barberry is very useful for many liver malfunctions including the ones caused by poor diet, medications or drugs.

Nutrition

The lack of nutrients in the diet, or the lack of a balance diet, can contribute to the discoloration of the area under the eyes. Vitamin and mineral deficiency are a very common cause of dark circles.

While researching for this report I notice that people from India a pre dispose to developing dark circles and I wanted to know the reason. It turns out that India's population is vegetarian due to religious beliefs, (cows are venerated animals). By digging deeper into their live styles, I found that Iron deficiency is the most pervasive of all nutritional deficiencies in India, particularly affecting women, especially pregnant women, as well as infants, young children and adolescent girls. Various estimates from different parts of the country indicate that more than 70% of pregnant women, approximately 50% of all women and 65-70% of adolescent girls may suffer from IDA Iron Deficiency Anemia. This brought me to the conclusion that Iron deficiency is one of the most common and important cause of dark circles under eyes.

A good, well balanced, healthy diet is essential for treating dark circles; but knowing how to eat a well-balanced diet is the hard part.

The numbers given by the Nutrition Board are a recommendation as to what Americans should be eating and how much in order to maintain their health. These recommendations are broken down into genders and age groups. For example, The RDA for a male fifty years of age is not the same as the RDA for a female 20 years of age.

RDAs are distinct from, but related to, the Reference Daily Intake (RDI) developed by the Food and Drug Administration to be used in food labeling. RDI replaced the term U.S. Recommended Daily Allowances which was used until new food labeling regulations went into effect in late 1992. All packaged foods were required to bear the new term on labels as of May 1994.
Because RDAs and RDIs are widely used, it is important to understand generally how to interpret them. The recommended allowances for nutrients are amounts intended to be consumed as part of a normal diet and are neither minimum requirements nor optimal levels of intake; it is not possible based on current research to set such specific guidelines nor to set a specific amount that would apply to all individuals. Rather, RDAs are safe and adequate levels of intake that reflect current knowledge.

Unfortunately most people don't eat well, not even the recommended amounts, this is the main cause of deficiency. Experts believe that many of the diseases affecting the average person are the result of not taking the necessary amount of nutrients needed to maintain a good health.

The problem is the complexity of the RDA table, for example, a child between 0 and 5 years of age needs 375 mg. of vitamin A, 7.5 mg. of vitamin D, 3 mg. of vitamin E, 5 mg. of vitamin K, 30 mg. of vitamin C, etc, etc, etc. and that's only for ages 0 - 5. As you can see there is no way to tell how much Vitamin D your child is taking a day or how much Iron is in the chicken your child had for lunch. The same problem is found in the RDA tables for men and women.

That is why I recommend the use of another method. The best way to know if you are getting the Recommended Dietary Allowance (RDA) for all the nutrients you need is to follow the Food guide pyramid. It provides from 1600 to over 2800 calories per day depending on which foods and the number of servings you eat. The assumption is made that if you will choose a variety of foods from each of the 5 food groups (Grain, Vegetable, Fruit, Milk, Meat) then you will probably get 100% of your RDA.

The Food Guide Pyramid is a tool used to teach people to eat a balanced diet from a variety of food portions without counting calories or any other nutrient. The USDA expanded the four food groups to six and expanded the number of servings to meet the calorie needs of most persons.

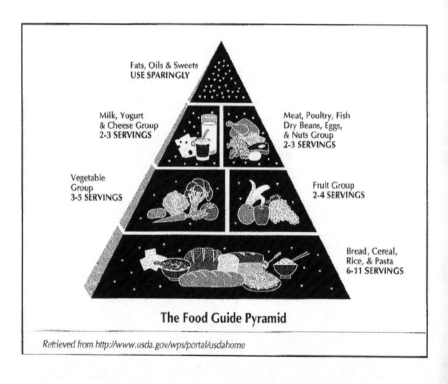

The Food Guide Pyramid

The Top of the Pyramid

Fats, oils and sweets should be used sparingly in the diet and therefore are represented as the small tip of the pyramid. This includes salad dressings, oils, cream, butter, margarine, soft drinks, candies and sweet desserts. These foods provide calories but little or no vitamins and minerals.

The Middle of the Pyramid

Protein is needed in moderate amounts in the diet and therefore represents the upper middle of the pyramid. Milk, yogurt, cheese, meat, poultry, fish, dry beans, eggs and nuts - two groups of foods that come mostly from animals - are important for protein, calcium, iron and zinc. Choose lean meats, skinless poultry, fish and low-fat dairy products to control fat and cholesterol. Also, limit breaded or fried foods to control fat and calories.

Most Americans need to eat more fruits and vegetables which helps form the foundation of the pyramid. Besides being an excellent source of vitamins, minerals and fiber, vegetables and fruits (plant foods) are low-fat, low-sodium and cholesterol-free.
Eating a variety of vegetables and fruits will help ensure that you meet your daily need for Vitamin C and other nutrients.

The Base of the Pyramid

Bread, cereals, rice and pasta - all foods from grains - are found at the base of the Pyramid because they are the foundation upon which the rest of the diet is planned. Try to choose 6-11 servings daily. Grains supply fiber, carbohydrates, vitamins and minerals. They are usually low in fat and are the preferred fuel for our brain, nervous system and muscles. To keep these foods low in fat and calories, limit the use of spreads.

The information in this brochure was adapted from USDA's Food Guide Pyramid, US Department of Agriculture, Human Nutrition Information Service, 1992.

What Counts as One Serving?

Here are some serving size examples for each food group. If you eat a larger portion, count it as more than one serving.

Most Americans are encouraged to eat at least the lowest number of servings from the five food groups each day.

Bread, Cereal, Rice and Pasta Group (6-11 servings)

1 slide of bread

• 1 ounce of ready-to-eat cereal (check labels: 1 ounce = 1/4 cup to 2 cups depending on cereal)

• 1/2 cup of cooked cereal, rice or pasta

• 1/2 hamburger roll, bagel, English muffin

• 3 or 4 plain crackers (small)

Vegetable Group (3-5 servings)

• 1 cup of raw leafy vegetables

• 1/2 cup of other vegetables, cooked or chopped raw

• 3/4 cup of vegetable juice

Fruit Group (2-4)

• 1 medium apple, banana, orange, nectarine, peach

• 1/2 cup of chopped, cooked or canned fruit

• 3/4 cup of fruit juice

Milk, Yogurt, and Cheese Group (2-3 servings)

- 1 cup of milk or yogurt

- 1.5 ounces of natural cheese

- 2 ounces of processed cheese

Meat, Poultry, Fish, Dry Beans, Eggs, and Nuts Group (2-3 servings)

- 2 to 3 ounces of cooked lean meat, poultry or fish

- (1 ounce of meat = 1/2 cup of cooked dry beans, 1 egg or 2 tablespoons of peanut butter)

How Much Should I Eat?

1200 calories is the lowest amount recommended to maintain nutritional adequacy; this calorie level is conducive for weight loss or extremely inactive individuals.

1600 calories is recommended for many sedentary women and some older adults.

2200 calories is recommended for most children, teenage girls, active women and sedentary men; women who are pregnant or breast feeding may need more.

2500 calories is recommended for teenage boys, active men and some very active women.

Important Note:
Remember that some of the foods recommended here my increase your chances of developing dark circles under the eyes, If you suffer from any type of food allergy you should avoid these foods, in such case a good multivitamin supplement could help you ingest the amount of nutrient you are missing out from your diet.

One more thing to take into account is to reduce the intake of dairy products, we already mention that these foods can contribute to dark circles and they should be reduced. I recommend eliminating dairy products completely from your diet for three weeks, if after this period you notice an improvement in you dark circles you should extend the period to two months, by then your dark circles will be drastically reduced then you can start incorporating to your diet, one dairy product every three days, always paying attention to how your

body accepts each food. If you noticed that your dark circles start to return after incorporating a particular dairy product you should remove it from your diet and replace it with a supplement that provides the nutrients contained in the dairy product you are unable to ingest.

FATIGUE, LACK OF SLEEP

This is an easy to tackle problem and a very important as well, because even if you are affected by any other condition that is causing your dark circles you can help reduce them by getting a good night sleep and resting at least eight hours. A lack of sleep or excessive tiredness can cause paleness of the skin, which again allows the blood underneath the skin to become more visible and appear more blue or darker.

Many people turn to sleeping pills for help but this is hardly the answer to insomnia problems. These drugs cause a number of side effects including liver damage, high blood pressure and they weaken the immune system. Besides, one can very easily become dependent of them. Once they do, a higher dose is needed and when they are discontinued the use withdrawal symptoms become a major problem and insomnia resumes along with agitation and fogginess which causes people to reach for the pills again and in an even higher dose. We are sure you will see that there is no need to put your body through pain caused by the side effects of these drugs, especially when there is a better answer in the form of natural herbs. Take a look.

We recommend

• Hops calms nerves, relieves tension and helps in cases of insomnia caused by stress, headaches and indigestion. It does not affect the early waking hours of the morning.

• A few hours before bedtime take Kava kava. It reduces stress, tension, anxiety and relaxes muscles. It helps you to fall asleep deeper and to rest more.   It can be used as a sedative when taking a large dose as effectively as benzodiazepines but without the side effects.

• The most popular herb for insomnia is Valerian. It relaxes nerves and muscles, improves sleep quality and makes falling asleep easier. Great for insomnia caused by mind activity, fear, fatigue or excitement. It's as good as many barbiturates but has no side effects or addiction.

Mix the following ingredients:
1 tsp. chamomile flowers.
1 tsp. hops.
1 tsp. valerian root.
1 cup of boiling water.
Steep for 45 minutes, strain and drink 1 hour before bedtime.

Make a tea mixing the following ingredients:
1 tbsp. of catnip leaves.
½ tbsp. of hops.
1 tbsp. of chamomile flower.
1 tbsp. of passionflower.
2 cups of boiling water.
Steep for 45 minutes, strain and drink 1 cup before bedtime.

• Catnip has sedative and tranquilizing properties. It is very good for insomnia caused by indigestion, gas, infant colic or menstrual cramps. It relaxes the body and mind during colds and flu.

• Passionflower helps if insomnia occurs from overwork, stress, pain, cough, drugs or alcohol. This is a great herb for children and infants teething, stomach pain etc. It soothes and relieves anxiety, irritability and is good for people with asthma or heart disease.

• Skullcap relieves insomnia caused by anxiety, worry or pain.

• Before going to bed, eat any of the following: bananas, milk, tuna, turkey and yogurt all of these contain tryptophan, it's been proven that they promote sleep.

• Avoid the following foods before bedtime: ham, cheese, chocolate, sausage, tomatoes and sugar.

• Do not use the bedroom for reading, watch TV, needle work etc. Go to the bedroom when you are sleepy or to for sex only.

• Jamaican dogwood is a strong pain reliever, sedative and antispasmodic. It's very helpful for muscular back pain, asthma, menstrual pain, insomnia, toothaches, and nervous conditions.

TIP: Did you know that waking up at 1:00 to 3:00 a.m. is a sign of a liver dysfunction?

MENSTRUATION

The skin can become paler during menstruation, which allows the underlying veins under the eyes to become more visible.

Women who experience severe premenstrual symptoms are far more likely to develop dark circles under their eyes. If you suffer from PMS certainly you have also notice dark circles under your eyes.

Premenstrual syndrome is the most common gynecological complaint of women and it affects about 60% of them. The symptoms appear one or two weeks before menstruation starts, and they include: abdominal bloating and cramps, acne, anxiety, breast tenderness and swelling and mood changes.

During menstruation there is an imbalance in hormones and brain activity and it is believed that too much estrogen, uneven levels of progesterone and an inability to cope with hormone changes are the main causes of PMS. But the real reason as to why this condition affects so many women is unknown.

About 5% of women suffer such severe complications that they are incapable of functioning normally during this period. Others claim symptoms interfere with their daily activities.

Using herbs we can return hormone levels to their normal level and proper diet can help reduce many of the symptoms. The final result is a body that is back in balance without using drugs and without experiencing any side effects.

We recommend

- Take magnesium 1,000 mg. a day. Deficiencies have been linked to PMS.

- Take calcium 1,500 mg. a day to help reduce some symptoms. Calcium and Magnesium combination.

- Take Vitamin B6 to reduce water retention and increase blood circulation to the female organs.

- Take Vitamin E to help reduce breast soreness.

TIP: Did you know that caffeine makes the changes of suffering from severe PMS symptoms 4 times greater?

- Black cohosh relieves premenstrual tension, menstrual cramps and water retention and helps control mood changes.

- Dandelion root is a very powerful diuretic that helps evacuate excess water and bloating but is safer then commercial diuretics because it does not deplete potassium. Another important quality is that it helps the liver discard estrogen thus relieving PMS.

- Dong Quai reduces cramps, pain and mood changes and regulates phytoestrogen leveling the hormones.

- Maca regulates hormones according to the body's need. It reduces acne occurrences and contains minerals and vitamins needed during PMS.

- Wild yam regulates levels of estrogen and progesterone. It relaxes the muscles and nerves.

- Studies have shown that Chaste tree regulates hormonal changes, reduces anxiety, mood changes and water retention and breast pain.

Mix the following ingredients:
1 tsp. of black cohosh root.
1 tsp. of passionflower.
1 tsp. of oregon grape root.
1 tsp. white willow bark.
2 cup of water.
Boil for 30 minutes, strain, take one tbsp. per hour.

Make a tea mixing:

1 tsp. black haw.
1 tsp. licorice root.
1 tsp. evening primrose.
1 tsp. milk thistle.
4 cups of boiling water.
Let it steep for 30 minutes, strain, drink 2 cups a day.

Mix the following ingredients
1 tsp. vitex berries.
1 tsp. wild yam rhizome.
½ tsp. burdock root.
½ tsp. dandelion root.
4 cups of boiling water.
Steep for 30 minutes, strain and drink 1 or 2 cups a day.

• Jamaican dogwood is a strong pain reliever, sedative and anti-spasmodic. Very helpful for muscular back pain, asthma, menstrual pain, insomnia, toothaches and nervous conditions.

Relaxing PMS Remedy
1 tsp. Valerian rhizome tincture.
½ tsp. catnip leaves tincture.
½ tsp. passionflower leaves tincture.
1/4 tsp. peppermint leaves tincture.
Mix all ingredients and take a dropperful 4 times a day.

Menstrual cramp oil

2 ounces Saint John's Wart oil.
8 drops Lavander essential oil.
8 drops Marjoram essential oil.
8 drops Chamomile essential oil.
Mix all ingredients and rub the lower abdomen with it as needed. This

formula can be used for back pain or any muscle related cramp.

Menstrual bleeding control tincture

1 tsp. shepherd's purse leaf tincture.
1 tsp. yarrow leaf tincture.
1/2 tsp. red raspberry leaf tincture.
1/2 tsp. vitex berry tincture.
Mix all ingredients and take 1/2 a dropperful 4 times a day.

Three other causes

The above causes are the ones everybody will tell you about when you ask the question what causes dark circles under the eyes? But here are three other reasons not many people know about (we will deal with all of them later):

Kidneys.
Heart.
Liver.

IMPORTANT TIP:

If the dark circles are black they are being caused by the kidneys.

If the dark circles are purple they are being caused by the heart.

If the dark circles are green they are being cause by the liver.

1. - KIDNEYS:

Although the kidneys are small organs by weight, they receive a huge amount – 20 percent -- of the blood pumped by the heart. The large blood supply to your kidneys enables them to do the following tasks.

• Regulate the composition of your blood

• Keep the concentrations of various ions and other important substances constant

• Keep the volume of water in your body constant

• Remove wastes from your body (urea, ammonia, drugs and toxic substances)

• Keep the acid/base concentration of your blood constant.

• Help regulate your blood pressure

• Stimulate the making of red blood cells

• Maintain your body's calcium levels

Your kidneys receive the blood from the renal artery, process it, return the processed blood to the body through the renal vein and remove the wastes and other unwanted substances in the urine. Urine flows from the kidneys through the ureters to the bladder. In the bladder, the urine is stored until it is excreted from the body through the urethra.

If your kidneys are not functioning properly toxins find their way back to the blood stream, the blood turns darker and since the capillaries in the eye area are small and numerous, the dark color becomes very noticeable.

Cleaning you kidneys is essential to remove dark circles under the eyes, if you suspect that you are having kidney deficiency problems, please consult with your doctor about using the following natural remedies.

• Celery and parsley are natural diuretics. Taken in combination, they are especially helpful if high uric acid levels are present in the blood. Eating large amounts of animal proteins makes one susceptible to high levels of uric acid. These two herbs help keep them in check.

• Cranberries contain substances that acidify the urine, destroy bacteria buildup and promote healing of the bladder. Drink 8 ounces of cranberry juice three times a day. Use pure unsweetened juice. If you don't like cranberry juice you can buy cranberry capsules.

• Dandelion root extract aids in excretion of the kidney's waste products.

• Uva ursi helps flush the kidneys and is also germicidal; if there are bacteria in the kidneys this herb will destroy them.

• Marshmallow tea cleanses the kidneys. Drink 3 cups a day.

• Eat a diet plentiful in raw vegetables and fruits including all of the following: Parsley, watermelon, juniper berries, bananas, asparagus, potatoes, cucumbers, garlic, papaya and most green vegetables.

• Make a tea mixing watermelon seeds and pumpkin seeds.

• Drink steam-distilled water.

- Punarnava is a weed. Its roots have incredible properties for kidney problems, especially because it rejuvenates nephron cells. Punarnava has anti-inflammatory and diuretic properties.

- Reduce your intake of the following: eggs, fish, meat, chocolate, beet greens, spinach and regular tea.

- Drink 4 glasses of raw goat's milk at body temperature every day. Add ¼ tablespoon of crude black-strap molasses to each glass.

- Take vitamin E and A.

TIP: Did you know that high doses of painkillers ibuprofen (Advil, Nuprin and others) can lead to kidney dysfunction.

Homemade Urinary Tonic

½ tsp. dandelion root,
½ oat straw,
½ nettle leaves,
½ rose hips,
¼ tsp. fennel,
¼ marshmallow root
1 quart of water.
Put herbs in water and bring to a simmer. Turn off heat and steep for 30 minutes. Strain and store in the refrigerator. Drink 2 cups a day.

Diuretic Tea

1 quart boiling water.
2 tsp. dandelion root,
½ tsp. nettle leaves,
½ tsp. oat straw,
½ tsp. fennel seed
½ tsp. corn silk.
Pour boiling water over herbs and then steep in a covered container for 30 minutes. Drink 1 cup a day.

2.-HEART:

Everyone knows that the heart is a vital organ. We cannot live without our heart. However, when you get right down to it, the heart is just a pump, a complex and important one, yes, but still just a pump. As with all other pumps it can become clogged, break down and need repair. This is why it is critical that we know how the heart works. With a little knowledge about your heart and what is good or bad for it, you can significantly reduce your risk for heart disease.

The heart, blood and blood vessels make up the system that supplies the body's tissues and organs with oxygen and nutrients.
Oxygen-depleted blood comes from all parts of the body to the chambers on the right side of the heart. The blood is then pumped through the lungs, where oxygen is added to it.
Oxygen-rich blood returns from the lungs to the left side of the heart and is pumped out, delivering oxygen to all the body's tissues.
If for some reason the heart pumps blood that is not sufficiently oxygenated, the blood turns darker and like in the kidneys case the color of the darker blood shows through the skin in the eye area.
However, I don't consider the heart as the most responsible for dark circles, although it cannot be ruled out.

In my opinion one of the less likely causes for your dark circles under your eyes could be the heart.

3. - LIVER:

The liver is an organ located on the right side of the body underneath the lower ribcage.

It is connected to the gallbladder and is involved in the absorption of fats and fat-soluble vitamins.

Blood carrying contents of the stomach and intestines flows directly to the liver, because the liver has a large role in protecting the body from harmful substances.

The liver is also integral to countless other metabolic processes. It produces more proteins than any other organ in the body.

- Stores and Mobilizes Energy

- Controls Blood Sugar (Glucose)

- Regulates Glycogen

- Regulates Fat Storage

- Aids Digestion

- Produces Bile

- Regulates Blood Clotting

- Manufactures

- Clotting Factors

- Other Blood Proteins

- Produces Several (Non-Reproductive) Hormones

Manufactures Cholesterol (a certain amount of cholesterol is beneficial)

- Filters Blood

- Eliminates Bacteria

- Detoxifies Poisons

- Externally-Derived Poisons

- Alcohol

- Byproducts of Metabolism

- Bilirubin

- Breaks down Drugs

- Produces Vitamins

- Vitamin D

- Stores Minerals

- Iron

- Produces Essential Immune System Factors

Monitors, as Well as Manufactures, Countless other Blood Proteins, to Maintain the Proper Levels of Numerous Chemicals in the Body.

Some or all the above mentioned functions can become impaired if the liver is congested, toxic and/or sluggish. Unfortunately this is very common in a majority of people, causing liver malfunctions.

Dark circles under the eyes are one of the first signs of liver problems and should be taken very seriously.

Liver Remedies for Dark Circles under Eyes

- Celandine it's a great herb for detoxification of the liver.

- Curcumin has shown incredible properties for reducing liver inflammation; it also protects the liver from toxic damage and increases bile flow.

- Dandelion it's a very important liver detoxifier, clearing wastes and pollutants.

- Milk thistle promotes regeneration and repair of liver tissue. It detoxifies and protects against damage by toxins and alcohol. Silymarin (milk thistle extract) has been shown in scientific studies to repair and rejuvenate the liver. Take 200 milligrams of silymarin 3 times a day.

- Barberry it's very useful for many liver malfunctions including the ones caused by poor diet, medications or drugs.

- Alfalfa helps build a healthy digestive tract and is a good source of vitamin K.

- Include the following to your diet: almonds, raw goat's milk grains and seeds.

- Do not drink alcohol, including over the counter medicines containing propylene glycol which is a form of alcohol.

- Eliminate the following from your diet: candies, milk, pepper, salt, spices, caffeine, colas, white rice, sugar, spicy and fried foods.

- Do not smoke and avoid second hand smoke.

Liver Tea

1 tsp. dandelion root.
1 tsp. milk thistle seeds.
1 tsp. roasted chicory root.
½ tsp. sarsaparilla root.
½ licorice root.
½ ginger rhizome.
1 quart water.
Combine ingredients in a sauce pan and simmer for a few minutes. Turn down heat and let steep for about 15 minutes. Strain and drink at least a cup a day.

Your Gallbladder is also involved

The gallbladder is a 3 to 4 inch-long pear-shaped organ located on the right side of the body, directly under the liver. One of the functions of the liver is to remove poisonous substance from the blood so that they can be excreted from the body. The liver excretes all these gathered toxins in a digestive agent called bile. Bile also contains cholesterol, bile salts, lecithin and other substances. The bile (about one pint of it every day) goes first to the gallbladder, which holds it until food arrives in the small intestine. The gallbladder then releases the bile, which passes through cystic and bile ducts into the small intestine. Ultimately, the toxins are passed out of the body through the feces. If your gallbladder is not doing its job, the liver has to work even harder which can cause liver problems as well.

I must insist that your liver is one of the keep factors in developing dark circles under your eyes, please follow some of the remedies below to treat and rejuvenate your gallbladder.

• Alfalfa cleanses the liver and supplies necessary vitamins and minerals. Twice a day for two days, take 1,000 milligrams in tablet or capsule form with a glass of warm water.

- Peppermint capsules are used in Europe to cleanse the gallbladder.

- If you have gallstones, or are prone to developing them, turmeric can reduce your risk of further problems.

- Other beneficial herbs include barberry root bark, catnip, cramp bark, dandelion, fennel, ginger root, horsetail, parsley and wild yam. **DO NOT USE BARBERRY DURING PREGNANCY.**

- If you have an attack, drink 1 tablespoon of apple cider in a glass of apple juice. This should relieve the pain quickly. If the pain does not subside, go to the emergency room to rule out other disorders such as gastroesophogeal reflux disease or heart problems.

- For inflammation of the gallbladder, don't eat solid food for a few days. Consume only distilled or spring water. Then drink juices such as pear, beet and apple for three days. Then add solid foods: shredded raw beets with 2 tablespoons of olive oil, fresh lemon juice, freshly made uncooked applesauce made in a blender or food processor. Apple juice aids in softening gallstones.

- For gallstones, take 3 tablespoons of olive oil with the juice of a lemon before bed and upon awakening. Stones are often passed and eliminated in the stool with this technique.

- Eat a diet that contains 75 percent raw foods. Include in the diet applesauce, eggs, yogurt, cottage cheese, broiled fish, fresh apples and beets.

- To cleanse the system drink as much apple juice as possible for five days. Beet juices also cleanse the liver.

- Avoid sugar and products containing sugar. People who consume an excessive amount of sugar are much more likely to form gallstones. Avoid all animal fat and meat, saturated fats, like chocolate, fried foods, soft drinks, spicy foods and full-fat dairy products.

Common Home remedies for dark circles

The remedies listed below are the ones most people know about, some of them are very useful if you have a very mild case of dark circles.

- Drink at least ten glasses of water every day.

- Eight hours of sleep is a must for all of us, especially for people having dark circles under their eyes.

- Close your eyes and cover your eyelids with slices of raw potato or cucumber for 15-20 minutes. Wash with warm water and apply a cream.

- Grate a cucumber, squeeze to take out its juice and refrigerate. Make a mixture of lemon juice, lanolin cream and cucumber juice and apply around the eye for 10-15 minutes.

- Apply lemon juice on the black circles 2 times a day.

- Apply a paste of turmeric powder with pineapple juice for dark circles under the eyes.

- Apply crushed mint around the eye.

- Apply almond oil under eyes.

- Almond helps to remove dark circles and is an excellent "skin food". Remove the cream applied around the eye after 10 min. No cream should be left on the skin around the eyes for long periods.

- Rub the area with a powdered Vitamin E capsule. And wipe off with a mixture of honey and egg white.

Chamomile is great for stress relief, if the dark circles under your eyes are due to stress and/or fatigue, drinking a cup of chamomile tea before you go to bed, it should help you relax.

Alternatively, steep the tea bag (unused) in cold mineral water for a few minutes. Soak a couple of cotton wool balls in the water, squeeze out the excess and place them over your closed eyelids for ten minutes.

You can now purchase chamomile sticks for treating the dark circles under your eyes. These can be carried with you and used as needed.

Dark Circles clearing poultice

Make a paste out of:
1 tsp. tomato juice,
1/2 tsp. lemon juice,
A pinch of turmeric powder
1 tsp. of flour.
Apply around eyes. Leave on for 10 minutes before rinsing.

Extract potato juice and cucumber juice in equal amounts. Soak cotton wool in this and apply around the eyes. It eliminates dark circles and refreshes the eyes.
Dark circles under eye paste.

Peel and chop a cucumber. Put it into a blender (add a little water if needed) and puree and refrigerate. Place over your eyes and lay down.

Five Day Dark Circles Remover Paste

During my research I found many herbs that help remove dark circles some with extraordinary result. Using my experience and the herbs that provided me the best outcome I created a recipe to treat dark circles. This recipe must be used in combination with the remedies for your underlying condition causing dark circles. I must insists on this to make it perfectly clear, this paste by itself will give you some result but it is the combine effect that makes this recipe a complete success.

This is the must have remedy, along with all the other remedies you have picked up from this e-book to remove your dark circles make sure you prepare this one, the herbs and essential oils can be found in most health and herbal stores. This recipe has shown me and the people whom have tried it unbelievable results. You should not take this one lightly.

There are five specialized herbs and two essential oils in this paste-

Ginseng,
Papaya,
Neem,
Pepermint,

Aswagandha (Withania Somniferra),
Sandalwood essential oil,
Almond essential oil.

Additionally:
Cucumber gel or Aloe Vera gel is added to prepare the paste.

Each ingredient has one or more specific property but it is the combination of all these herbs and oils that contributes towards the end result.

Preparation:
Buy the herbs in powder form, you can also buy the capsules and open them to make the preparation or get the herbs and coffee grinder them. Mix 3 teaspoons of each powdered herb. Add 3 drops of each essential oil. Add cucumber gel or Aloe Vera gel, enough to make a paste. Apply under your eyes for 30 minutes twice a day.

The Immune System and its role in dark circles

Sixty five years ago medical scientists promised us that infections caused by bacteria and others would be a thing of the past due to the new discovery of patented pharmaceutical drugs. This very brave statement was made and almost automatically more than half of the herbs recommended in the U.S. Pharmacopoeia were taken off to be replaced with these chemical drugs. I wish I could tell you that the promised was kept and that now we live in an infection free world, but this is not so. We are all familiar with the enormous amounts and resistance of bacteria. Antibiotics have not live up to their promised; to the contrary they have become a problem in itself, by over use and side effects that cause liver, kidney, nervous and immune system damage.

Modern conventional medicine battles diseases directly by means of drugs, surgery, radiation and other therapies, but true health can be attained only by maintaining a healthy properly functioning immune system.

It is the immune system that fights off disease-causing microorganisms and it engineers the healing process. The immune system is the key to fighting every kind of insult to the body, from that little shaving scratch to the gigantic amount of viruses the constantly try to invade our bodies. Even the aging process may be related to a deteriorated immune system.

Weakening of the immune system makes us vulnerable to every type of illness that affects humans. Some common signs of impaired immune functions include fatigue, lassitude, repeated infections, inflammation, allergic reactions, slow wound healing, chronic diarrhea and infections related to overgrowth of benign organisms already present in the body, such as oral thrush, vaginal yeast infections and other fungal infections. It is calculated that a normal adult gets an average of two colds per year. People suffering from colds more than the average are likely to have some sort of immune deficiency. Dark circles could be directly related to an immune system malfunction.

Explaining what the immune system is the hard part. The immune system it is not an organ but an interaction between many organs, structures and substances with the task of recognizing or differencing from things that belong and those that don't belong to the body, and then neutralizing or destroying the ones that are foreign.

The immune system is like no other bodily system, the patrolling and protecting tasks of the immune system are share by white cells, bone marrow, the lymphatic vessels and organs, specialized cells found and various body tissues, and specialized substances, called serum factors, that are present in the blood. Ideally, all of these components work together to protects the body against diseases.

To boost and protect your immune system I recommend a list of herbs, vitamins, supplements and special recipes that have shown remarkable results throughout the years.

Astragalus boosts the immune system and generates anticancer cells in the body. It is also a powerful antioxidant and protects the liver from toxins. This makes this plant ideal for people suffering from dark circles due to liver problems and depressed immune system. IMPORTANT: Do not take this herb if fever is present.

Baybarry has antibiotic effects for sore throat, coughs, clods and flu. Garlic is effective against at least 30 types of bacteria, viruses, parasites and fungi. It has anti-inflammatory and astringent properties.

Echinacea boosts the immune system and enhances lymphatic function.

Goldenseal strengthens the immune system, cleanses and detoxifies the body. It has anti bacteria properties.

In a small town called Chirchik, Russia, a flu epidemic swept the town. When many adults and children did not get sick scientists wanted to know why they were immune to the disease. It turns out that all of them used the berries from an herb called Shizandra.

Immune System Booster

2 cups of water.
1 tsp. echinacea root.
½ tsp. chamomile leaves.
½ tsp. shizandra berries.
½ tsp. peppermint leaves.

Immune Tincture.

½ tsp. Echinacea root tincture.
½ tsp. pau d´arco bark tincture.
½ tsp. Siberian ginseng root tincture.
½ tsp. licorice root tincture.
½ tsp. astragalus root tincture.
½ tsp. bupleurum root tincture.
Combine all these ingredients. If you have evidence of a depressed immune system, take 3 tsp. of the formula daily for up to 5 days. Double the dose during an infection.

Include in the diet chlorella, garlic and pearl barley. These foods contain germanium, a trace element beneficial for the immune system. Also giant red kelp contains iodine, calcium, iron, carotene, protein, riboflavin and vitamin C, which are necessary for the immune system's functional integrity.

Vitamin C may be the single most important nutrient for the immune system. It is essential for the formation of adrenal hormones and the production of lymphocytes. It also has direct effect on bacteria and viruses. Vitamin C should be taken with bioflavonoids, natural plant substances that enhance absorption and reinforce the action of this vitamin.

The "Do not Do this" List for Dark Circles under the Eyes

Do not drink caffeine especially at night time.

Do not wash your face with hot water.

Do not take aspirin:
It is very common for many people to drink a cup of coffee (caffeine) in the morning and take an aspirin. Aspirin thins blood which many wrongly believe that prevents heart problems; the problem is that aspirin also kills red blood cells, which carry oxygen plasma into the blood.

Don't eat too much dairy products:
Some people are sensitive to dairy products and the do develop dark circles under the eyes. This might be related to some kind of food allergy.

Do not drink sodas:
Sodas contain sugar and caffeine which is harmful for people with severe dark circles.

Do not take Vitamin A in excess:
Excess vitamin A or an overdose of Retin-A is very likely to cause liver problems, which can cause dark circles under eyes.

Do not eat sugar:
Sugar is the enemy for people suffering severe dark circles. Research about the action of insulin shows that sugar can lead not only to weight problems, but also skin problems, through inflammatory responses as well as their effect on protein which can age the skin and the body prematurely through a process called glycation. Inflammation leads to eye puffiness.

Do not eat salty foods:
Cut down by half your daily intake of salt. Salt produces fluid
retention this increases the pressure in the small capillaries in your
eye area aggravating your dark circles.

Complications of Dermatologic Laser Surgery

One of the answers I got the most while researching a cure for dark
circles was that laser surgery was nearly the only treatment with
optimal result, and a 100% success rate. Well this is hardly the entire
truth about laser treatments.

The popularity of dermatologic laser surgery has skyrocketed in the
past decade, as have the number of indications for its use and the
types of lasers. As with all surgical modalities, excellent results are
tempered by complications.

When laser light hits the skin, it may be reflected, transmitted, or
absorbed. Absorbed energy is most responsible for the clinical effect
because it is converted to thermal energy by absorption of heat by
the intended targets. In many cases, complications result from
collateral damage created when energy intended for the target
chromophore is not selectively diffused to and absorbed by
surrounding tissue. For example, hyperpigmentation and
hypopigmentation noted after carbon dioxide laser resurfacing are
related to damage to cells in the basal layer of the epidermis
vaporized along with targeted cells in the epidermis and dermis.

Carbon dioxide laser has been a popular surgeon's tool over the past
several years to remove dark circles under the eyes, but its use has
been limited due to the risk of scarring and pigment changes
resulting from the deep thermal damage (or heat build-up) it
produces in the skin. Complications include milia formation, perioral
dermatitis, acne and/or rosacea exacerbation, contact dermatitis, and
postinflammatory hyperpigmentation. Moderate complications include
localized viral, bacterial, and candidal infection, delayed

hypopigmentation, persistent erythema, and prolonged healing. The most severe complications are hypertrophic scarring, disseminated infection, and ectropion. Early detection of complications and rapid institution of appropriate therapy are extremely important. Delay in treatment can have severe deleterious consequences, including permanent scarring and dyspigmentation.

Erythema is an acute mucocutaneous hypersensitivity reaction of variable severity characterized by a symmetrically distributed skin eruption, with or without lesions in some cases, prolonged erythema that may persist for several months. Of greater concern is the potential for delayed permanent hypopigmentation seen in as many as 20% of patients when multiple-pass carbon dioxide resurfacing is performed.

A laser procedure to remove dark circles can cost you $100 for 15 minutes of treatment, but usually it will take more than one treatment to get an acceptable result. Laser treatment is very expensive and it may carry some undesired side effects.

I'm sure that after reading this information you will think twice before undergoing laser surgery to remove dark circles and I hope this section of the report helps you make a better decision when it comes to dark circle removal and laser treatment.

Resources

The herbs and minerals used in this report to treat dark circles are listed below in a convenient alphabetical order to help you learn more about each individual herb and mineral. Refer to this list to see all the properties and studies done.

This list will also assist you in determining what other uses these plants have, as we all know any herb and mineral is beneficial in many different conditions.

There is a long list of herbs that when used as shown in this report will help vanish dark circles from your face, please make sure you follow the steps described in the report for optimum results.

Alfalfa (Medicago sativa)
Alfalfa has been used by the Chinese since the sixth century to treat kidney stones and to relieve fluid retention and swelling. It is a perennial herb that grows throughout the world in a variety of climates. Alfalfa grows to about 3 feet and has blue- violet flowers that bloom from July to September.
First discovered by the Arabs, they dubbed this valuable plant the "father of all foods". They fed alfalfa to their horses claiming it made the animals swift and strong. The leaves of the alfalfa plant are rich in

minerals and nutrients, including calcium, magnesium, potassium and carotene (useful against both heart disease and cancer). Leaf tablets are also rich in protein, vitamins E and K. Alfalfa extract is used by food makers as a source of chlorophyll and carotene.

The leaves of this remarkable legume contain eight essential amino acids. Alfalfa is a good laxative and a natural diuretic. It is useful in the treatment of urinary tract infections and kidney, bladder and prostate disorders. Alkalizes and detoxifies the body, especially the liver. Promotes pituitary gland function and contains an anti-fungus agent.

Part Used: Whole herb and leaf.

Common use: This versatile herb is also a folk remedy for arthritis, diabetes, asthma, hay fever and is reputed to be an excellent appetite stimulant and overall tonic. Excellent source of nutritive properties with minerals, chlorophyll and vitamins. Alfalfa is high in chlorophyll and nutrients. Treating with alfalfa preparations is generally without side effects; however the seeds contain a slightly toxic amino acid L-canavanine.

Aloe (Aloe vera)

Aloe, native to Africa, is also known as "lily of the desert", the "plant of immortality" and the "medicine plant". The name was derived from the Arabic alloeh meaning "bitter" because of the bitter liquid found in the leaves. In 1500 B.C. Egyptians recorded use of the herbal plant in treating burns, infections and parasites.

There are over 500 species of aloe growing in climates worldwide. Ancient Greeks, Arabs and Spaniards have used the plant throughout the millennia. African hunters still rub the gel on their bodies to reduce perspiration and their scent.

Extensive research since the 1930's has shown that the clear gel has a dramatic ability to heal wounds, ulcers and burns by putting a protective coating on the affected areas and speeding up the healing rate.

The plant is about 96% water. The rest of it contains active

ingredients including essential oil, amino acids, minerals, vitamins, enzymes and glycoproteins. Modern healers have used it since the 1930's. Many liquid health treatments are made, some combining aloe juice with other plants and herbs. The juice is soothing to digestive tract irritations, such as colitis and peptic ulcers.
As a food supplement, aloe is said to facilitate digestion, aid in blood and lymphatic circulation, as well as kidney, liver and gall bladder functions.

Aloe contains at least three anti-inflammatory fatty acids that are helpful for the stomach, small intestine and colon. It naturally alkalizes digestive juices to prevent overacidity - a common cause of indigestion. It helps cleanse the digestive tract by exerting a soothing, balancing effect.
A newly discovered compound in aloe, acemannan, is currently being studied for its ability to strengthen the body's natural resistance. Studies have shown acemannan to boost T-lymphocyte cells that aid the immune system.

Those wise to the ways of aloe healing keep this plant in the kitchen. When the leaf is broken, its gel is placed on burns to relieve pain and prevent blisters. Aloe may reduce inflammation, decrease swelling and redness and accelerate wound healing.
Aloe can aid in keeping the skin supple and has been used in the control of acne and eczema. It can relieve itching due to insect bites and allergies. Aloe's healing power come from increasing the availability of oxygen to the skin and by increasing the synthesis and strength of tissue.

Part Used: Aloe vera "extract" is made by pulverizing the whole leaves of the plant. Aloe juice is made from the inner leaf.

Common Use: Aloe supplements can be used for peptic ulcers and for gastro-intestinal health. Aloe has a moisturizing effect on the skin and is a common remedy for sunburn and skin irritation. Often used direct form the flowerpot in the treatment of minor burns and wounds. To make a salve; remove the thin outer skin and process the leaves in a blender, add 500 units of vitamin C powder to each cup and store in refrigerator.

Bearberry or Uva ursi:
In consequence of the powerful astringency of the leaves, Uva-Ursi has a place not only in all the old herbals, but also in the modern Pharmacopoeias.
The usual form of administration is in the form of an infusion, which has a soothing as well as an astringent effect and marked diuretic action. Of great value in diseases of the bladder and kidneys, strengthening and imparting tone to the urinary passages. The diuretic action is due to the glucoside Arbutin, which is largely absorbed, unchanged and is excreted by the kidneys. During its excretion, Arbutin exercises an antiseptic effect on the urinary mucous membrane: Bearberry leaves are, therefore, used in inflammatory diseases of the urinary tract, urethritis, cystitis, etc.

Cat's Claw (Uncaria tomentosa)
Cat's Claw is a tropical vine that grows in rainforest and jungle areas in South America and Asia. Some cultures refer to the plant as the "Sacred Herb of the Rain Forest". This vine gets its name from the small thorns at the base of the leaves, which looks like a cat's claw. These claws enable the vine to attach itself around trees climbing to heights up to 100 feet.

The plant is considered a valuable medicinal resource and is protected in Peru. Although scientific research has just recently begun to explore cat's claw, many cultures native to the South American rain forest areas have used this herb for hundreds of years.
Current studies show it may have positive effects on and can boost the body's immune system. With recent fear of HIV, studies on cat's claw have started to move quickly.

The active substances in Cat's Claw are alkaloids, tannins and several other phytochemicals. Some of the alkaloids have been proven to boost the immune system. The major alkaloid rhynchophylline has anti-hypertensive effects and may reduce the risk of stroke and heart attack by lowering blood pressure, increasing circulation, reducing heart rate and controlling cholesterol.

Other constituents contribute anti-inflammatory, antioxidant and anticancer properties. Many treatments combine the herb with different plants and natural products to increase the absorption and bioavailability.

Cat's Claw has long been used as a homeopathic treatment for intestinal ailments. Uses include: Crohn's disease, gastric ulcers and tumors, parasites, colitis, gastritis, diverticulitis and leaky bowel syndrome. By stimulating the immune system, it can also improve response to viral and respiratory infections.
European clinical studies have used the extract from the bark in combination with AZT in the treatment of AIDS. It is also used in the treatment and prevention of arthritis and rheumatism, as well as diabetes, PMS, chronic fatigue syndrome, lupus and prostrate conditions.

Part Used: Inner bark and root. Capsules, tea and extract.

Common Use: Extracts are used in treatments for a variety of conditions, mostly gastrointestinal. Immune-stimulant properties help the body fight off infections and protect against degenerative diseases.

Chaste Tree

DANDELION TARAXACUM OFFICINALE
This herb helps one to see farther without a pair of spectacles. This is known by foreign physicians who are not so selfish as ours, but more communicative of the virtues of plants to people. A well-known plant which barely requires description. It is known to the vulgar as Piss-a-Beds, which is due no doubt to its diuretic property. The root grows down exceedingly deep and if broken off within the ground it will shoot forth again.

Where to find it: A troublesome weed all over the world in meadows, pastures and gardens. Flowering time: Throughout the year.

Medicinal virtues: It has an opening and cleansing quality and, therefore, very effectual for removing obstructions of the liver, gall bladder and spleen and diseases arising from them, such as jaundice. It opens the passages of the urine both in young and old and will cleanse ulcers in the urinary tract. For this purpose the decoction of the roots or leaves in white wine, or the leaves used as pot herbs are very effectual. It is of wonderful help in cachexia, the severe wasting condition in severe illness. It also procures rest and sleep in those with fever. The distilled water can be drunk in pestilential fever and he used as a wash for the sores. This common herb hath many virtues, which is why the French and Dutch eat them so often in the spring.

Modern uses: Bile production by the liver and urinary output from the kidneys is increased with the use of this herb. As a diuretic, it is superior to many produced synthetically by pharmaceutical companies. The leaves are particularly strong, being equivalent to frusemide, a drug used to treat hypertension. The dried herb contains significant amounts of potassium, which people on long-term diuretic therapy need. Modern herbalists, therefore, have a safe, but powerful remedy, not only for hypertension but also for cardiac oedema, hepatogenic dropsy and water retention, due to stasis or congestion in the blood vessels serving the liver.

The diuretic effect of Dandelion is helpful in the treatment of a number of other conditions, particularly chronic disorders like rheumatisrn, gout and eczema. A fluid extract is available from herbalists and the recommended dose is between one and two teaspoonfuls three times a day. The dried root taken in the form of a decoction is a powerful liver tonic - 1 oz. (28 g) of the root is boiled in 2 pt (1.1 l) of water until the mixture is reduced to 1 pt. (568 rnl). The dose is two to four teaspoonful three or four times a day. A Dandelion coffee made from the roasted roots is available from health stores. The fresh, clean young leaves can be added to salads in spring.

Don Quai (Angelica sinensis)

Dong quai is an aromatic herb that grows in China, Korea and Japan. The reputation of Don quai is second only to Ginseng and is considered the ultimate, all-purpose woman's tonic herb. It is used for almost every gynecological complaint from regulating the menstrual cycle to treating menopausal symptoms caused by hormonal changes.

Dong quai is frequently used by the Chinese as a strengthening treatment for the heart, spleen, liver and kidneys. Both men and women use the herb as a general blood tonic.

Dong quai contains vitamins E, A and B12. Researchers have isolated at least six coumarin derivatives that exert antispasmodic and vasodilatory effects. Antispasmodics are a remedy for menstrual cramps. The essential oil in dong quai contains Ligustilide, butylphthalide and numerous other minor components. Ferulic acid and various polysaccharides are also found in dong quai's root. These elements can prevent spasms, reduce blood clotting and relax peripheral blood vessels. Research has shown that don quai produces a balancing effect on estrogen activity.

Modern treatments prescribe the herb to combat PMS and to help women resume normal menstruation after using birth control pills.

The herb has been found useful in balancing and treating many female systems and cycles. Dong quai's constituents can act to stimulate the central nervous system which can remedy weakness and headaches associated with menstrual disorders. It strengthens internal reproductive organs, helps with endometriosis and internal bleeding or bruising. It relieves menopausal conditions such as vaginal dryness and hot flashes.
The herb has also been used as a blood purifier, to promote blood circulation and nourish the blood in both sexes. It is high in iron content and may help to prevent iron deficiency and anemia. Studies show that it can aid in regulating blood sugar and in lowering blood pressure.

Dong quai has a mild sedative effect which can relieve stress and calms the nerves. It has also be used to stimulate the uterus during childbirth, treat insomnia, alleviate constipation and for migraine headaches.

Parts Used: Whole root. Found in tea, herbal preparations, capsules, extract and recipes.

Common Use: The root has earned a reputation as the "ultimate herb" for women. It is used to restore balance to a woman's hormones and cycles and is helpful in restoring menstrual regularity and for conditions of the reproductive system. It is not recommended during pregnancy, for women with excessive menstrual flow or for people taking blood thinning agents.

Echinacea (Echinacea angustifolio)

Resembling a black-eyed Susan, Echinacea or purple coneflower is a North American perennial that is indigenous to the central plains where it grows on road banks, prairies, fields and in dry, open woods. It is also called snake root because it grows from a thick black root that Indians used to treat snake bites.

Herbalists consider Echinacea one of the best blood purifiers and an effective antibiotic. It activates the body's immune system increasing the chances of fighting off any disease. This popular herb has been used to help ward off the common cold and to relieve the symptoms of hay fever.

The Plains Indians used various species of Echinacea to treat poisonous insect and snake bites, toothaches, sore throat, wounds, as well as mumps, smallpox and measles. The settlers quickly adopted the therapeutic use of the plant and since that time it has become one of the top selling herbs in the United States. Since the early 1900's many of scientific articles have been written about Echinacea. Most of the research during the past 10 years has focused on the immunostimulant properties of the plant.

The constituents of Echinacea include essential oil, polysaccharides, polyacetylenes, betain, glycoside, sesquiterpenes and caryophylene. It also contains copper, iron, tannins, protein, fatty acids and vitamins A, C and E. The most important immune-stimulating components are the large polysaccharides, such as inulin, that increase the production of T-cells and increase other natural killer cell activity. Fat-soluble alkylamides and a caffeic acid glycoside called echinacoside also contribute to the herb's immune empowering effects.

It has been shown in animal and human studies to improve the migration of white blood cells to attack foreign microorganisms and toxins in the bloodstream. Research suggests that echinacea's activity in the blood may have value in the defense of tumor cells.

Echinacea properties may offer benefit for nearly all infectious conditions. Studies show echinacea prevents the formation of an enzyme which destroys a natural barrier between healthy tissue and damaging organisms. Echinacea is considered an effective therapeutic agent in many infectious conditions including upper respiratory infections, the common cold and sinusitis. The herb is a mild antibiotic that is effective against staph and strep infections.

Echinacea aids in the production of interferon have increases antiviral activity against, influenza (flu), herpes, an inflammation of the skin and mouth. It may reduce the severity of symptoms such as runny nose and sore throat and reduce the duration of illness.
Echinacea's antibacterial properties can stimulate wound healing and are of benefit to skin conditions such as burns, insect bites, ulcers, psoriasis, acne and eczema. Its anti-inflammatory properties may relieve arthritis and lymphatic swelling.

It has also been used in homeopathy treatments for chronic fatigue syndrome, indigestion, gastroenteritis and weight loss.
Part Used: Root, dried; also liquid extract and juice. It is often used in combination with goldenseal or vitamin C.

Common Use: Echinacea products are used as a general nonspecific stimulant to the immune system, supporting and stabilizing cellular immunity and cleansing the blood, for the prevention and treatment of infections. There are no known side effects associated with its use.

Folic Acid:
A series of recent studies suggest that this B vitamin may be a major player in warding off heart attacks, strokes and certain common cancers. Often called folacin or folate (its biologically active form), it also is well established as critically important in the prevention of

birth defects of the brain and spinal cord, called neural tube defects, if taken before pregnancy and in the first few weeks of pregnancy.. The following foods contain significant quantities of folic acid: Barley, beef, bran, brewer's yeast, brown rice, cheese, chicken, dates, green leafy vegetables, lamb, legumes, liver, milk, mushrooms, oranges, split peas, pork, root vegetables, salmon, tuna, wheat germ, whole grains, whole wheat. TIP: A sore, red tongue is one sign of folic acid deficiency.

Garlic (Allium sativum)
Garlic is a member of the onion family and is nature's most versatile medicinal plant. Garlic has been used all over the world for thousands of years for a wide range of conditions. It has been prized since the first records of civilization for its uses in treating wounds, infections, tumors and intestinal parasites.

Modern scientists in numerous clinical trials have concluded that Garlic lowers cholesterol, lowers blood pressure, thins the blood (which reduces your risk of heart attack and stroke) and fights bacteria like an antibiotic.

Garlic is a potent antioxidant that has been found to inhibit tumor cell formation and is currently being studied by the National Cancer Institute. It may be effective in fighting stomach, skin and colon cancer.

Though it is best known as a culinary herb and vampire retardant, the medicinal benefits and claims for garlic have awarded it the name "Wonder Drug among all herbs".

Modern day research helps explain the broad applications of this "miracle" herb. Garlic bulbs contain the amino acid allicin. When crushed, allicin is released. This chemical element is the component that gives Garlic its strong odor and is responsible for the powerful pharmacological properties of the plant. One medium clove of Garlic can equal the antibacterial action equivalent to 1% penicillin.

Garlic also contains about 0.5% of a volatile oil that is composed of sulfur-containing compounds. Garlic's sulfur compounds, in addition to Selenium and Vitamins A and C containing compounds, make it a potent antioxidant, protecting cell membranes and DNA from damage and disease.

Although Garlic directly attacks bacteria and viruses, it also stimulates the body's natural defenses against foreign invaders.

Garlic is reported to be more effective than penicillin against typhus disease and works well against strep, staph bacteria and the organisms responsible for cholera, dysentery and enteritis.
It is generally regarded as a preventative measure for colds, flu and other infectious diseases. Furthermore, scientific studies have shown that garlic stimulates the production of the liver's own detoxifying enzymes which neutralize carcinogens and other environmental toxins. It has also been used to rid the body of intestinal parasites and to treat digestive infections.

Researchers have been studying the anti-cancer properties of Garlic since the 1940's. It appears that the herb may prevent cells from turning cancerous by enhancing the body's mechanisms for removing toxic substances. Garlic's phytochemicals are believed to enhance immunity and the National Cancer Institute (January 1992) reported that people who ate the greatest amount of onions and garlic had the lowest incidence of stomach cancer. Other types of cancer have also been reported as lower.

Furthermore, garlic increases the activity of white blood cells and T-helper cells (natural killer cells), the cells that are central to the activity of the entire immune system.

Garlic supplements can improve many of the processes that can lead to cardiovascular disease. Garlic has been used as a blood thinner and anticoagulant to resolve blood clots and improve circulation. It has been shown to lower cholesterol while increasing the level of beneficial HDLs (high-density lipoproteins), the so-called good cholesterol.

Garlic has no side effects like those associated with cholesterol lowering drugs. (Take garlic for at least two or three months, as often in the first month or two, cholesterol may actually slightly rise.) In addition, garlic compounds gently lower blood pressure by slowing the production of the body's own blood pressure raising hormones. At least seventeen clinical trials have shown that mild hypertension can be effectively managed with garlic.

Garlic has great value as a long-term dietary supplement, helping to maintain healthy circulation, balance blood sugar and pressure, reduce fat levels in the blood and improve resistance to infection. It can be taken with conventional antibiotics to support their action and ward off side effects.

Garlic has also been used in treating upper respiratory infections (especially bronchitis), late-onset diabetes, urinary infections, acne, asthma, sinusitis, arthritis and ulcers.

Part Used: Bulb or as odorless tablets.

Common Use: Good for virtually any disease or infection. Improves circulation, maintains healthy cholesterol and blood pressure levels. It is a natural antibiotic and immune system stimulant.

Ginseng (Panax ginseng)
Ginseng is the most famous Chinese herb. It is the most widely recognized plant used in traditional medicine. Various forms of ginseng have been used in medicine for more than 7000 years. Several species grow around the world and though some are preferred for specific benefits, all are considered to have similar properties as an effective general rejuvenator.
The name panax is derived from the Greek word panacea meaning, "all healing" and the benefits of ginseng are recognized as such.

Ginseng is commonly used as an adaptogen, meaning it normalizes physical functioning depending on what the individual needs (for example, it will lower high blood pressure, but raise low blood pressure).

It is also used to reduce the effects of stress, improve performance, boost energy levels, enhance memory and stimulate the immune system. Oriental medicine has deemed ginseng a necessary element in all their best prescriptions and regards it as prevention and a cure.

It is said to remove both mental and bodily fatigue, cure pulmonary complaints, dissolve tumors and reduce the effects of age.

Ginseng is native to China, Russia, North Korea, Japan and some areas of North America. It was first cultivated in the United States in the late 1800's. It is difficult to grow and takes 4-6 years to become mature enough to harvest. The roots are called Jin-chen, meaning 'like a man,' in reference to their resemblance to the shape of the human body.

Native North Americans considered it one of their most sacred herbs and add it to many herbal formulas to make them more potent. The roots can live for over 100 years.

Ginseng contains vitamins A, B-6 and the mineral Zinc, which aids in the production of thymic hormones, necessary for the functioning of the defense system. The main active ingredients of ginseng are the more than 25 saponin triterpenoid glycosides called "ginsenosides". These steroid-like ingredients provide the adaptogenic properties that enable ginseng to balance and counter the effects of stress. The glycosides appear to act on the adrenal glands, helping to prevent adrenal hypertrophy and excess corticosteroid production in response to physical, chemical or biological stress.

Studies done in China showed that ginsenosides also increase protein synthesis and activity of neurotransmitters in the brain. Ginseng is used to restore memory and enhance concentration and cognitive abilities, which may be impaired by improper blood supply to the brain.

Ginseng helps to maintain excellent body functions. Siberian ginseng has been shown to increase energy, stamina and help the body resist viral infections and environmental toxins. Research has shown specific effects that support the central nervous system, liver function, lung function and circulatory system.

Animal studies have shown that ginseng extracts stimulate the production of interferons, increase natural killer cell activity, lower cholesterol and decrease triglyceride levels. Men have used the herb to improve sexual function and remedy impotence. Ginseng is believed to increase estrogen levels in women and is used to treat menopausal symptoms.

It is also used for diabetes, radiation and chemotherapy protection, colds, chest problems, to aid in sleep and to stimulate the appetite.

Part used: Whole root. Powdered in capsules, as an ingredient in many herbal formulas and as a tea.

Common Use: Ginseng is one of the most popular healing herbs used today throughout the world. It increases mental and physical efficiency and resistance to stress and disease. Ginseng's adaptogenic qualities help balance the body, depending on the individual's needs. It is known to normalize blood pressure, increase blood circulation and aid in the prevention of heart disease.

Ginkgo Biloba
Sadly, in America, medicine and health are a big business so the properties of this tree are not publicized. Europeans have come to rely on Ginkgo extract to treat many illnesses. In Germany and France it's been registered as a drug and it's one of the most commonly prescribed remedies. In Germany Ginkgo has been authorized for the treatment of a wide array of cerebral problems, ranging from ringing in the ears, to memory loss, anxiety, headaches, dizziness and nervousness. It has been approved to treat circulatory disorders as well. Latest research done in Germany and France has shown extremely good results using Ginkgo Biloba extract to treat Alzheimer's, even reversing the disease when caught early.

The main property of Ginkgo is its ability to improve circulation to all parts of the body, including the brain. This is believed to be a key benefit to Alzheimer's and stroke patients. By improving blood flow Ginkgo helps the body deliver essential nutrients and oxygen to damaged areas of the body. Ginkgo nourishes blood vessels which decreases the chances of heart attacks and circulatory problems.

Another property of Ginkgo is the ability to fight free radicals (see antioxidants). Due to its antioxidant characteristics Ginkgo searches for free radicals, attacking them and leaving harmless molecules in their place.

Goldenseal (Hydrastis canadenis)
Goldenseal is a Native American medicinal plant introduced to early settlers by Cherokee Indians who used it as a wash for skin diseases, wounds and for sore, inflamed eyes. Its roots are bright yellow, thus the name. Goldenseal root has acquired a considerable reputation as a natural antibiotic and as a remedy for various gastric and genitourinary disorders.

Numerous references to Goldenseal began to appear in medical writings as far back as 1820 as a strong tea for indigestion. Today it is used to treat symptoms of the cold and flu and as an astringent, antibacterial remedy for the mucous membranes of the body. This popular North American herb grows wild in moist mountainous woodland areas. Goldenseal's long history of use among North Americans flourished after the Civil War as it was an ingredient in many patent medicines. It has been collected to the point of near extinction. Goldenseal supplies are diminishing and most is now wild crafted, making herbal supplements costly.

Goldenseal is used in many combination formulas and is reported to enhance the potency of other herbs. Preparations have been marketed for the treatment of menstrual disorders, urinary infections, rheumatic and muscular pain and as an antispasmodic. The active ingredients in Goldenseal are the alkaloids hydrastine and berberine. Similar in action, they destroy many types of bacterial and viral infections. These alkaloids can also reduce gastric inflammation and relieve congestion. Berberine is a bitter that aids digestion and that has a sedative action on the central nervous system. Goldenseal works wonders in combination with Echinacea particularly at the onset of cold and flu symptoms, especially coughs and sore throats. Goldenseal, Echinacea and Zinc lozenges should be in every medicine cabinet.

Goldenseal is a cure-all type of herb that strengthens the immune system, acts as an antibiotic, has anti-inflammatory and antibacterial properties, potentiates insulin and cleanses vital organs. It promotes the functioning capacity of the heart, the lymphatic and respiratory system, the liver, the spleen, the pancreas and the colon.

Taken internally, Goldenseal increases digestive secretions, astringes the mucous membranes that line the gut and checks inflammation. It also aids digestion by promoting the production of saliva, bile and other digestive enzymes. In addition it may control heavy menstrual and postpartum bleeding by means of its astringent action.

As a dilute infusion, Goldenseal can be used as eyewash and as a mouthwash for gum disease and canker sores. It is also an effective wash or douche for yeast infections. External applications have been used in the treatment of skin disorders such as psoriasis, eczema, athlete's foot, herpes and ringworm.

Part Used: Whole root.

Common Use: Treatment of any infection, inflammation and congestion of lungs, throat and sinuses. It's Famous for use in treatment of cold and flu. It is a potent remedy for disorders of the stomach and intestines such as irritable bowel syndrome, colitis, ulcers and gastritis and internal parasites.

Cautions: The use of very large doses can or extended use is not suggested. Not for use during pregnancy or by children under two. Children and older adults should take smaller doses.

Horse Chestnut:
The bark has tonic, narcotic and febrifuge properties and is used in intermittent fevers, given in an infusion as an external application to ulcers; this infusion has also been used with success.

The fruits have been employed in the treatment of rheumatism and neuralgia and also in rectal complaints and for hemorrhoids.

The plant is taken in small doses internally for the treatment of a wide range of venous diseases, including hardening of the arteries, varicose veins, phlebitis, leg ulcers, hemorrhoids and frostbite. It is also made into a lotion or gel for external application. Horse chestnut is an astringent, anti-inflammatory herb that helps to tone the vein walls. The bark is anti-inflammatory, astringent, diuretic, febrifuge, narcotic, tonic and vaso-constrictive.

Licorice (Glycyrrhiza glabra)
Licorice is a perennial herb native to southern Europe, Asia and the Mediterranean. It is extensively cultivated in Russia, Spain, Iran and India. It is one of the most popular and widely consumed herbs in the world.

Although many know this herb for its flavoring in candy, licorice contains many health benefits. Ancient cultures on every continent have used licorice, the first recorded use by the Egyptians in the 3rd century BC. The Egyptians and the Greeks recognized the herb's benefits in treating coughs and lung disease. Licorice is the second most prescribed herb in China followed by ginseng, it is suggested for treatment of the spleen, liver and kidney. The Japanese use a licorice preparation to treat hepatitis.

The most common medical use for licorice is for treating upper respiratory ailments including coughs, hoarseness, sore throat and bronchitis.

The main constituent found in the root is glycyrrhizin. The plant also contains various sugars (to 14%), starches (30%), flavonoids, saponoids, sterols, amino acids, gums and essential oil. Glycyrrhizin, stimulates the secretion of the adrenal cortex hormone aldosterone.

It can be as effective as codeine and safer, when used as a cough suppressant. Rhizomes in licorice have high mucilage content which, when mixed with water or used in cough drops, sooths irritated mucous membranes. The drug also has an expectorant effect which increases the secretion of the bronchial glands. Licorice is an effective remedy for throat irritations, lung congestion and bronchitis.

Homeopathic use of licorice for gastric irritation dates back to the first century. Today, herbal preparations are used to treat stomach and intestinal ulcers, lower acid levels and coat the stomach wall with a protective gel. Rarely used alone, it is a common component of many herbal teas as mild laxative, a diuretic and for flatulence. It has also been known to relieve rheumatism and arthritis, regulate low blood sugar and is effective for Addison's disease. The root extract produces mild estrogenic effects and it has proven useful in treating symptoms of menopause, regulating menstruation and relieving menstrual cramps.

The main ingredient glycyrrhizin has also been studied for its anti-viral properties in the treatment of AIDS. In clinical trials in Japan it prevented progression of the HIV virus by inhibiting cell infection and inducing interferon activity. Glycyrrhizin also encourages the production of hormones such as hydrocortisone which give it anti-inflammatory properties. Like cortisone it can relieve arthritic and allergy symptoms, without the side effects.

The constituent glycyrrhizin is 50 times sweeter than sugar, making it a widely used ingredient in the food industry. The distinctive flavor of licorice makes it a popular additive to baked confections, liqueurs, ice cream and candies. It is also widely used in other medicines to mask bitter tastes and also to prevent pills from sticking together.

Licorice has also been used in poultices for treatment of dermatitis and skin infections. It helps to open the pores and is used in combination with other cleansing and healing herbs as an emollient. Part Used: Root in the making of powder, teas and tonics, extracts, tinctures and decoctions.

Common Use: It is an ingredient in many cough medicines and a popular and well-known remedy for bronchial distress. It can have a beneficial effect on gastric disturbances.

Milk Thistle (Silybum marianus)
This plant is native to the Mediterranean and grows wild throughout Europe, North America and Australia. Milk Thistle has been used in Europe as a remedy for liver problems for thousands of years. Its use was recorded in the first century (AD 23-79), noting that the plant was excellent for protecting the liver. Early Christian tradition dedicated milk thistle to Mary, calling it Marian thistle. In the 19th century the Eclectics used the herb for varicose veins, menstrual difficulty and congestion in the liver, spleen and kidneys. Milk thistle has also been taken to increase breast-milk production, stimulate the secretion of bile and as a treatment for depression.

Milk thistle nutritionally supports the liver's ability to maintain normal liver function. It has shown positive effects in treating nearly every known form of liver disease, including cirrhosis, hepatitis, necroses and liver damage due to drug and alcohol abuse. Milk thistle works due to its ability to inhibit the factors responsible for liver damage, coupled with the fact it stimulates production of new liver cells to replace old damaged ones.

Milk thistle has been proven to protect the liver from damage. The detrimental effects of environmental toxins, alcohol, drugs and chemotherapy may be countered with this valuable herb. The active chemical component in the herb is silybin, which functions as an antioxidant and is one of the most potent liver protective agents known. Clinical trials have proven silybin to be effective in treating chronic liver diseases and in protecting the liver from toxic chemicals.

An injection of silybin is a proven antidote for poisoning with the Deathcap mushroom (Amanita phalloides).
Silybin is a part of the chemical structure of the flavoligan silymarine. Milk thistle's hepatoprotective effects may be explained by its function of altering the liver cell membrane structure, blocking the absorption of toxins into the cells. Hepatoprotection by silymarin can also be attributed to its ability to increase the intracellular concentration of glutathione, a substance required for detoxicating reactions in liver cells. Milk thistle is also an antioxidant that is more potent than vitamins C and E.

Parts Used: Seeds for powdered or liquid extract.

Common Use: Helps the liver detoxification process. It helps for all liver disorders such as jaundice and hepatitis. Fights pollutants and prevents free radical damage by action as antioxidant. Protects the liver and stimulates the production of new liver cells. Helps common skin conditions related to poor liver function.

MSM methylsulfonylmethane, may help decrease an allergic reaction. Take 500milligrams 2 or 3 times a day.

Nettle:

Although not prescribed by the British Pharmacopoeia, the Nettle has still a reputation in herbal medicine and is regarded in homoeopathy as a useful remedy. Preparations of the herb have astringent properties and act also as a stimulating tonic.

Nettle is anti-asthmatic: the juice of the roots or leaves, mixed with honey or sugar, will relieve bronchial and asthmatic troubles and the dried leaves, burnt and inhaled, will have the same effect. The seeds have also been used in consumption, the infusion of herb or seeds being taken in wineglassful doses. The seeds and flowers used to be given in wine as a remedy for ague. The powdered seeds have been considered a cure for goiter and efficacious in reducing excessive corpulence. Preparations of Nettle are said to act well upon the kidneys, but it is a doubtful diuretic, though it has been claimed that incipient dropsy may be remedied by tea made from the roots.

Pantothenic acid, aid in the processing of food amino acids. They also support the function of the adrenal glands, which is important in the control of allergies. Click Here

Peppermint:

Peppermint oil is the most extensively used of all the volatile oils, both medicinally and commercially. The characteristic anti-spasmodic action of the volatile oil is more marked in this than in any other oil and greatly adds to its power of relieving pains arising in the alimentary canal.

From its stimulating, stomachic and carminative properties, it is valuable in certain forms of dyspepsia, being mostly used for flatulence and colic. It may also be employed for other sudden pains and for cramp in the abdomen; wide use is made of Peppermint in cholera and diarrhea.

It is generally combined with other medicines when its stomachic effects are required, being also employed with purgatives to prevent griping. Oil of Peppermint allays sickness and nausea and is much used to disguise the taste of unpalatable drugs, as it imparts its aromatic characteristics to whatever prescription it enters into.

Menthol is used in medicine to relieve the pain of rheumatism, neuralgia, throat affections and toothache. It acts also as a local anesthetic, vascular stimulant and disinfectant. For neuralgia, rheumatism and lumbago it is used in plasters and rubbed on the temples; it will frequently cure neuralgic headaches. It is inhaled for chest complaints and nasal catarrh. Laryngitis or bronchitis is often alleviated by it. It is also used internally as a stimulant or carminative. On account of its anesthetic effect on the nerve endings of the stomach, it is of use to prevent sea-sickness, the dose being 1/2 to 2 grains. The bruised fresh leaves of the plant will, if applied, relieve local pains and headache and in rheumatic affections the skin may be painted beneficially with the oil.

Primrose oil contains gamma-linolenic acid (GLA).

Punarnava:

Punarnava is a weed. Its roots help maintain efficient kidney and urinary functions with its diuretic, anti-spasmodic and anti-inflammatory action.
It helps kidneys, especially the rejuvenation of nephron cells.
Because of its mild diuretic properties it also helps in the treatment of obesity. In combination with other diuretics it also has a role in cardiac diseases; Punarnava has anti-inflammatory and diuretic properties.

Salmon resources Salmon capsules

St. John's Wort
St. John's wort is a bushy perennial plant with numerous yellow flowers. It is native to many parts of the world including Europe and the United States. It is a wild growing plant in northern California, southern Oregon and Colorado.

73

The plant has been used as an herbal remedy since the middle Ages.

It has a 2,400-year history of safe and effective usage in many folk and herbal remedies. Historically used as a nerve tonic, St. John's wort is now widely used as a mild antidepressant. It is a potent antiviral and antibacterial that is being investigated as a treatment for AIDS.

One of the best herbs for mood elevation is St. John's wort. Several controlled studies have shown positive results in treating patients with mild to moderate depression. Improvement was shown with symptoms of sadness, helplessness, hopelessness, anxiety, headache and exhaustion with no reported side effects.

Its action is based on the ability of the active ingredient, hypericin to inhibit the breakdown of neurotransmitters in the brain. The herb also inhibits monoamine oxidase (MAO) and works as a serotonin reuptake inhibitor (SRI); both are actions similar to drugs prescribed for depression. In Germany, nearly half of depression, anxiety and sleep disorders are treated with hypericin. St. John's wort should not be taken with any other antidepressants, it is not effective for severe depression and no one should stop taking any prescribed medications for depression without proper medical care.

St. John's wort has been administered in the treatment of many illnesses. The most well-known action of St. John's wort is in repairing nerve damage and reducing pain and inflammation. The herb has been used to relieve menstrual cramping, sciatica and arthritis. It has a favorable action on the secretion of bile and thus soothes the digestive system.

The blossoms have been used in folk medicine to relieve ulcers, gastritis, diarrhea and nausea. St. John's wort can also be effective in the treatment of incontinence and bed-wetting in children. Externally it is used on cuts as a disinfectant and to relieve inflammation and promote healing. The oil can be applied to sprains, bruises and varicose veins. Folk medicine has also has used it as a treatment for cancer.

The active constituents in the herb (there are over 50) include hypericin and pseudohypericin, flavonoids, tannins and procyanidins.

The tannins are responsible for the astringent effect for wound healing. Hypericin increases capillary blood flow and is a MAO inhibitor.

There are many studies documenting the clinical effects of hypericum as an antidepressant treatment similar to several synthetic antidepressants, but with a minimum of side effects. Hypericin has been demonstrated to increase theta waves in the brain. Theta waves normally occur during sleep and have been associated with deep meditation, serene pleasure and heightened creative activity. St. John's wort effectually may improve perception and clarify thinking processes.

There have been incidences of photosensitization as a side effect in animals. Anyone who is hypersensitive to sunlight or is taking other photosensitizing drugs should be cautious.

Parts Used: Herb tops and flowers. Used as a tea, extract, oil and in tablet form.

Common Use: St. John's wort has been used traditionally as an herbal treatment for anxiety and depression. It is an effective astringent that promotes wound healing and has antiviral properties that can counter herpes simplex, flu viruses and is being investigated as a treatment for acquired immunodeficiency syndrome (AIDS).

Note: If you are pregnant or lactating or taking anti-depressants like Prozac, check with your physician before taking St. John's wort. St. John's Wort is known to interfere with a number of prescription medications, including anticoagulants, oral contraceptives, antidepressants and anti-seizure medications, drugs to treat HIV or prevent transplant rejection. The above statements have not been evaluated by the FDA and are not intended to diagnose, treat, cure or prevent any disease.

Shark cartilage reduces inflammation.

SHILAJIT:

Over sixty years of clinical research have shown that shilajit has positive effects on humans. It increases longevity, improves memory and cognitive ability, reduces allergies and respiratory problems, reduces stress and relieves digestive troubles. It is anti-inflammatory, antioxidant and eliminates free radicals. The research proves that shilajit increases immunity, strength and endurance and lives up to its ancient reputation as the "destroyer of weakness."
Shilajit amplifies the benefits of other herbs by enhancing their bio-availability, helps transport nutrients deep into tissue and remove deep-seated toxins, improves memory and the ability to handle stress, reduces recovery time in muscle, bone and nerve injuries, stimulates the immune system and reduces chronic fatigue.

Turmeric

Turmeric is a tropical perennial of the ginger family that is native to India. Herbal preparations are derived from the plant's yellowish-orange root, which has also long been used as a dye. Turmeric is a prime component of curry powders and is used as a spice to flavor many types of food. It serves as a multipurpose herbal remedy for practitioners of Ayurveda, the traditional healing system of India and practitioners of traditional Chinese medicine. They recommend it as a digestive aid, a wound healer and a liver remedy. Only in recent years have herbalists elsewhere in the world begun to appreciate turmeric's therapeutic potential, as scientific studies confirm many of the traditional uses and suggest additional benefits such as protection from heart disease and cancer.

Turmeric has been used for thousands of years as an anti-inflammatory agent in the treatment of sprains, cramps, bruises and muscle pain. Topical applications have been used to promote the healing of wounds and skin conditions. In ancient times a potent household remedy was to make a poultice from turmeric mixed with slaked lime. Taken orally, turmeric is a favorite folk remedy for infections and parasites of the stomach and the intestines. Turmeric is a traditional remedy for jaundice and other liver ailments. Herbalists have also used turmeric to help treat diarrhea, fever, headaches, flatulence, bronchitis and colds and coughs.

Herbalists as well as an increasing number of doctors are now aware of the anti-inflammatory properties of turmeric root extracts. Turmeric may be as effective as cortisone for acute inflammation, though somewhat less so for chronic inflammation. Turmeric alleviates the pain of rheumatoid arthritis and prevents menstrual discomfort. Turmeric may also combat intestinal microbes. Its antioxidant properties may help to prevent cancer and protect the liver. Recent studies suggest turmeric can lower blood cholesterol levels and reduce the stickiness of blood platelets, thus decreasing the risk of stroke and heart attack in some people.

Vitamin B6

Vitamin C:
Vitamin C is an antioxidant that is required for tissue growth and repair, adrenal gland function and healthy gums. It also aids in the production of anti-stress hormone and interferon and is needed for metabolism of folic acid. It protects against the harmful effects of pollution, helps to prevent cancer, protects against infections and enhances immunity. Vitamin C increases the absorption of iron. It also may reduce cholesterol levels and high blood pressure. Protects against blood clotting and bruising and promotes the healing of wounds and burns.

Vitamin C is found in berries, citrus fruit and green vegetables. Good sources include asparagus, broccoli, Brussels sprouts, cantaloupe, dandelion greens, papayas, lemons, pineapple, strawberries and tomatoes. Herbs that contain vitamin C include alfalfa, burdock root, horsetail, peppermint and nettle.

Vitamin E:
Vitamin E is an antioxidant that is important in the prevention of cancer and cardiovascular disease. It improves circulation, necessary for tissue repair and is useful in treating premenstrual syndrome and fibrocystic disease of the breast. It promotes normal blood clotting and healing, reduces blood pressure; it also maintains healthy muscles while strengthening capillary walls.

Vitamin K:

Vitamin K is needed among other things for the production of prothrombin, which is necessary for blood clotting.   It is also essential for bone formation and repair; it is necessary for the synthesis of osteo-calcin, the protein in bone tissue on which calcium crystallizes. Consequently, it may help prevent osteoporosis.

Vitamin K plays an important role in the intestines and aids in converting glucose into glycogen for storage in the liver, promoting healthy liver function. A deficiency of this vitamin can cause internal bleeding.

Vitamin K is found in some foods, including asparagus, broccoli, Brussels sprout, cabbage, dark green leafy vegetables, liver, oatmeal, wheat. Herbs that contain vitamin k are: alfalfa, green tea and nettle.

Made in the USA
Middletown, DE
28 June 2016